INFLAMMATION INTERRUPTED

7 proven secrets to regulate your immune system and unlock optimal health

ESTHER C. EXCEL

Inflammation interrupted

Table of contents

INTRODUCTION

Welcome to Inflammation Interrupted: Igniting a Revolution Within

The Spark That Ignites Transformation

Imagine a life where energy and vitality flow effortlessly, where your body and mind thrive in harmony, and where the whispers of inflammation are silenced. This is the promise of Inflammation Interrupted, a journey that will revolutionize how you understand and interact with your body.

The Unseen Enemy

Inflammation is a master of disguise, masquerading as fatigue, pain, or weight gain. But beneath its subtle symptoms lies a complex web of biological responses that can either heal or harm. It's time to expose the truth about inflammation and reclaim your power.

A Personal Odyssey

As we embark on this journey together, I invite you to reflect on your own experiences with inflammation. What sparks your curiosity? What fuels your frustration? What whispers of hope still linger? Your story is unique, and it's time to rewrite the narrative.

Embracing the Unknown

Inflammation Interrupted is not a destination; it's a journey of discovery, exploration, and empowerment. It's an invitation to venture into the uncharted territories of your body and mind, to confront the unknown, and to emerge transformed.

Let the Journey Begin

In this moment, you stand at the threshold of a new chapter in your life. Please take a deep breath, and let's step into the unknown together.

PART 1:

UNDERSTANDING INFLAMMATION

Chapter 1: The Fire Within - What is Inflammation and Why Should You Care?

Inflammation: The Double-Edged Sword

Imagine a fire raging within your body, fueled by a complex mix of biological responses. This fire, known as inflammation, can be both a protector and a destroyer. It's a natural defense mechanism that heals wounds and fights off infections, but when left unchecked, it can ravage your body, leaving a trail of chronic diseases in its wake.

The Invisible Epidemic

Inflammation is the silent saboteur of modern life, quietly wreaking havoc on millions of people worldwide. It's the common thread linking chronic diseases like arthritis, diabetes, cardiovascular disease, and even mental health disorders. Yet, despite its pervasive impact, inflammation remains shrouded in mystery.

Unraveling the Mystery

To understand inflammation, we must venture into the intricate world of immune responses, cellular signaling, and molecular mechanisms. It's a fascinating journey that reveals the dynamic interplay between your body's defense systems and the environment.

Why You Should Care

Inflammation affects us all, either directly or indirectly. Its impact is felt in:

- Chronic pain and fatigue
- Weight gain and metabolic disorders

- Skin issues and aging
- Mental health and mood disorders
- Gut health and digestive issues

The Power of Knowledge

By grasping the fundamentals of inflammation, you'll unlock the secrets to:

- Preventing chronic diseases
- Optimizing your immune system
- Enhancing your overall wellbeing
- Taking control of your health

Embark on the Journey

As we delve deeper into the world of inflammation, remember that knowledge is power. Empower yourself to understand the fire within, and discover how to harness its energy to transform your life.

Chapter 2: The Immune System - Your Body's Defense Against Inflammation

The Guardian of Your Health

Imagine a highly trained army, strategically positioned within your body, ever-vigilant and ready to defend against invaders. This army is your immune system, a complex network of cells, tissues, and organs working in harmony to protect you from harm.

The Immune System's Dual Role

Your immune system plays a dual role in the inflammation saga. It's both the hero that saves the day and the villain that wreaks havoc. On one hand, it's responsible for triggering inflammation to fight off infections and heal wounds. On the other hand, an overactive or misdirected immune response can lead to chronic inflammation, causing more harm than good.

The Players in the Immune System

Meet the key players in your immune system's army:

- White blood cells (leukocytes): The soldiers that fight off infections
- Lymph nodes: The communication hubs that coordinate the immune response
- Spleen: The filter that removes pathogens and damaged cells
- Thymus: The training ground for immune cells
- Bone marrow: The factory that produces immune cells

The Immune Response

When your body detects a threat, the immune system springs into action:

1. Recognition: Identifying the invader
2. Activation: Triggering the immune response
3. Proliferation: Producing more immune cells
4. Resolution: Eliminating the threat and resolving inflammation

The Inflammation Connection

Inflammation is a natural byproduct of the immune response. Acute inflammation is a necessary response to injury or infection, but chronic inflammation arises when the immune system fails to resolve the response, leading to ongoing tissue damage.

Tipping the Balance

Factors that can disrupt the immune system's balance include:

- Genetics
- Environmental toxins
- Stress
- Poor diet

- Lack of sleep

Achieving Harmony

To maintain immune system harmony:

- Fuel your body with a balanced diet
- Stay hydrated
- Exercise regularly
- Manage stress
- Get enough sleep

The Power of Immune System Balance

By understanding your immune system and its role in inflammation, you'll unlock the secrets to:

- Boosting your immune function
- Preventing chronic diseases
- Enhancing your overall wellbeing
- Taking control of your health

Empower Yourself

As you continue on this journey, remember that knowledge is power. Empower yourself to understand your immune system and its intricate relationship with inflammation. By doing so, you'll become the master of your health destiny.

Chapter 3: The Gut-Inflammation Connection - How Your Microbiome Impacts Your Health

The Hidden World Within

Deep within your belly lies a vast, uncharted territory, home to trillions of microorganisms. This is your gut microbiome, a complex ecosystem that plays a crucial role in your overall health. The gut-inflammation connection is a fascinating story of how your microbiome influences your body's inflammatory response.

The Microbiome: A Delicate Balance

Your gut microbiome is a harmonious balance of beneficial and pathogenic microorganisms. When this balance is disrupted, the consequences can be far-reaching, leading to chronic inflammation and various diseases.

The Gut-Brain Axis

The gut and brain are intimately connected through the gut-brain axis. Your gut microbiome produces neurotransmitters and hormones that influence your mood, cognitive function, and overall well-being.

The Inflammation Link

Dysbiosis, an imbalance of the gut microbiome, triggers inflammation in several ways:

- Producing pro-inflammatory compounds
- Disrupting the gut barrier function
- Altering the immune response

The Consequences of Dysbiosis

An imbalanced gut microbiome has been linked to:

- Inflammatory bowel disease
- Obesity and metabolic disorders
- Mental health issues
- Autoimmune diseases
- Cardiovascular disease

Nourishing Your Microbiome

Feed your gut microbiome with:

- Fiber-rich foods
- Polyphenol-rich foods
- Omega-3 fatty acids
- Probiotics
- Prebiotics

Restoring Balance

To restore balance to your gut microbiome:

- Avoid antibiotics and antimicrobials
- Limit processed foods
- Manage stress

- Stay hydrated
- Exercise regularly

The Power of the Gut-Inflammation Connection

By understanding the intricate relationship between your gut microbiome and inflammation, you'll unlock the secrets to:

- Preventing chronic diseases
- Enhancing your immune function
- Boosting your mood and cognitive function
- Achieving optimal wellbeing

Embrace the Connection

As you continue on this journey, remember that your gut microbiome is a powerful ally in the fight against inflammation. By nurturing and balancing your microbiome, you'll unlock a world of possibilities for optimal health and well-being.

PART 2:

7 PROVEN SECRETS TO REGULATE YOUR IMMUNE SYSTEM

Chapter 4: Secret 1: Nutrition and Inflammation - The Foods That Fuel or Calm the Fire

The Power of Nutrition

Nutrition plays a crucial role in the inflammation saga. The foods you eat can either fan the flames of inflammation or help extinguish them. In this chapter, we'll explore the first secret to taming inflammation: nutrition.

The Pro-Inflammatory Foods

Some foods can trigger or exacerbate inflammation:

- Refined sugars
- Processed meats
- Dairy products
- Gluten-containing grains
- Fried foods
- Foods high in saturated and trans fats

The Anti-Inflammatory Foods

On the other hand, some foods have potent anti-inflammatory effects:

- Fatty fish (rich in omega-3s)
- Leafy greens (rich in antioxidants)
- Nuts and seeds (rich in healthy fats and antioxidants)
- Fruits (rich in antioxidants and fiber)
- Turmeric (contains curcumin)
- Ginger
- Olive oil

The Gut-Friendly Foods

A healthy gut microbiome is essential for reducing inflammation. Include gut-friendly foods in your diet:

- Fermented foods (kimchi, sauerkraut, kefir)
- Fiber-rich foods (legumes, whole grains, fruits)
- Polyphenol-rich foods (berries, green tea, dark chocolate)

The Inflammation-Reducing Nutrients

Certain nutrients have anti-inflammatory properties:

- Omega-3 fatty acids
- Antioxidants (vitamins C and E, beta-carotene)
- Polyphenols
- Probiotics
- Vitamin D

Creating Your Anti-Inflammatory Diet

To reduce inflammation through nutrition:

- Eat a balanced diet rich in whole foods
- Avoid pro-inflammatory foods
- Incorporate anti-inflammatory foods
- Stay hydrated
- Limit processed and packaged foods

The Power of Nutrition in Action

By making informed food choices, you can:

- Reduce chronic inflammation
- Improve your immune function
- Enhance your overall well being
- Increase your energy levels
- Support your mental health

Embrace the Nutrition Secret

By unlocking the first secret of nutrition and inflammation, you'll be empowered to take control of your health and well-being.

Remember, every bite counts, and the right foods can help calm the fire of inflammation.

Chapter 5: Secret 2: Stress Less, Live More - The Impact of Stress on Inflammation

The Silent Saboteur: Stress

Stress is a ubiquitous presence in modern life, and its impact on inflammation cannot be overstated. In this chapter, we'll delve into the second secret to taming inflammation: stress management.

The Stress-Inflammation Connection

Stress triggers a cascade of physiological responses, including:

- Release of pro-inflammatory cytokines
- Activation of immune cells
- Increased blood sugar levels

- Disruption of the gut microbiome

Chronic Stress: The Inflammation Catalyst

Chronic stress perpetuates inflammation, leading to:

- Insulin resistance
- Cardiovascular disease
- Mental health disorders
- Weakened immune function
- Skin issues

The Stress Response: Fight or Flight

The body's stress response is designed for short-term protection, but chronic activation leads to:

- Adrenal fatigue
- Hormonal imbalance
- Inflammation

Stress Management Techniques

Discover the power of:

- Mindfulness meditation
- Yoga
- Deep breathing exercises
- Progressive muscle relaxation
- Journaling
- Grounding techniques

The Relaxation Response

Activate the relaxation response to counteract stress:

- Reduce cortisol levels
- Increase oxytocin and dopamine
- Enhance immune function
- Promote gut health

Creating a Stress-Less Life

To reduce stress and inflammation:

- Prioritize self-care
- Set boundaries
- Engage in activities that bring joy
- Practice gratitude
- Seek social support

The Power of Stress Management

By embracing stress management techniques, you can:

- Reduce chronic inflammation
- Enhance your immune function
- Improve your mental health
- Increase your resilience
- Live a more balanced life

Embrace the Stress-Less Secret

By unlocking the second secret of stress management, you'll be empowered to break free from the cycle of chronic stress and inflammation. Remember, a stressless life is a more vibrant life.

Chapter 6: Secret 3: Move Your Body, Calm Your Inflammation - The Power of Excrcise

Unleash the Power of Movement

Exercise is a potent tool in the fight against inflammation. In this chapter, we'll explore the third secret to taming inflammation: movement.

The Exercise-Inflammation Connection

Regular exercise:

- Reduces pro-inflammatory cytokines
- Increases anti-inflammatory cytokines
- Enhances immune function
- Improves cardiovascular health
- Supports gut health

The Anti-Inflammatory Effects of Exercise

Exercise-induced benefits include:

- Reduced systemic inflammation
- Improved insulin sensitivity
- Enhanced mental health
- Increased muscle mass and strength
- Better sleep quality

The Science Behind Exercise and Inflammation

Understand the mechanisms:

- Muscle contraction and inflammation reduction
- Exercise-induced antioxidant production
- The role of myokines in inflammation regulation

Find Your Ideal Exercise Routine

Discover activities that bring you joy:

- Aerobic exercises (running, cycling, swimming)
- Resistance training (weightlifting, bodyweight)
- Flexibility exercises (yoga, Pilates)
- High-Intensity Interval Training (HIIT)
- Mind-body exercises (tai chi, qigong)

Creating a Movement Plan

To reduce inflammation through exercise:

- Start slow and progress gradually
- Aim for consistency and frequency
- Incorporate variety and fun
- Listen to your body and rest
- Seek professional guidance

The Power of Movement in Action

By embracing exercise, you can:

- Reduce chronic inflammation
- Improve your overall health
- Enhance your mental wellbeing

- Increase your energy levels
- Live a more vibrant life

Embrace the Movement Secret

By unlocking the third secret of movement, you'll be empowered to harness the power of exercise to calm inflammation and transform your life. Remember, every step counts, and movement is medicine.

Chapter 7: Secret 4: Sleep and Inflammation - The Restorative Power of a Good Night's Sleep

Sleep: The Unsung Hero

Sleep is a vital component of immune system regulation. In this chapter, we'll explore the fourth secret to taming inflammation: sleep.

The Sleep-Inflammation Connection

Sleep deprivation triggers:

- Increased pro-inflammatory cytokines
- Activation of immune cells
- Disrupted gut microbiome
- Impaired immune function

The Restorative Power of Sleep

Adequate sleep:

- Reduces inflammation
- Enhances immune function
- Supports gut health
- Regulates hormones
- Improves mental health

The Science Behind Sleep and Inflammation

Understand the mechanisms:

- Sleep's impact on cytokine regulation
- The role of sleep in immune cell function
- Sleep's effect on gut barrier function

Tips for a Restful Night's Sleep

Improve your sleep hygiene:

- Establish a consistent sleep schedule
- Create a sleep-conducive environment
- Avoid screens before bedtime

- Engage in relaxing activities
- Avoid stimulating activities before bedtime

The Power of Sleep in Action

By prioritizing sleep, you can:

- Reduce chronic inflammation
- Enhance your immune function
- Improve your mental wellbeing
- Increase your energy levels
- Live a more balanced life

Embrace the Sleep Secret

By unlocking the fourth secret of sleep, you'll be empowered to harness the restorative power of a good night's sleep to regulate your immune system and calm inflammation. Remember, sleep is not a luxury, it's a necessity.

Additionally, consider the following:

- Get 7-9 hours of sleep each night

- Practice relaxation techniques, like deep breathing or meditation, before bed
- Avoid caffeine and heavy meals close to bedtime
- Create a sleep diary to track your progress
- Seek professional help if sleep disorders persist

Chapter 8: Secret 5: Mindfulness and Meditation - Taming the Flames of Inflammation

The Mind-Body Connection

Mindfulness and meditation are powerful tools for regulating the immune system and reducing inflammation. In this chapter, we'll explore the fifth secret to taming inflammation: mindfulness and meditation.

The Impact of Stress on Inflammation

Chronic stress triggers inflammation, which can lead to various diseases. Mindfulness and meditation help mitigate stress, reduce inflammation, and promote overall well-being.

The Science Behind Mindfulness and Meditation

Understand the mechanisms:

- Reduced cortisol levels
- Increased anti-inflammatory cytokines
- Enhanced immune function
- Improved gut health
- Increased grey matter in the brain

Tips for Mindfulness and Meditation

Start your mindfulness journey:

- Begin with short sessions (5-10 minutes)
- Focus on breath, body, or emotions
- Practice mindfulness in daily activities
- Use guided meditations or apps
- Make mindfulness a habit

The Power of Mindfulness in Action

By incorporating mindfulness and meditation, you can:

- Reduce chronic inflammation
- Enhance your immune function
- Improve your mental wellbeing
- Increase your resilience
- Live a more balanced life

Embrace the Mindfulness Secret

By unlocking the fifth secret of mindfulness and meditation, you'll be empowered to tame the flames of inflammation and transform your life. Remember, mindfulness is a journey, not a destination.

Additionally, consider the following:

- Start small and be consistent
- Find a quiet and comfortable space for meditation
- Be patient and gentle with yourself
- Explore different types of meditation (loving-kindness, transcendental, etc.)
- Incorporate mindfulness into your daily routine

Chapter 9: Secret 6: Supplements and Inflammation - The Science-Backed Solutions

The Power of Supplements

While a balanced diet is essential, supplements can help bridge nutritional gaps and support immune function. In this chapter, we'll explore the sixth secret to taming inflammation: science-backed supplements.

The Science Behind Supplements and Inflammation

Understand the mechanisms:

- Omega-3 fatty acids: Reduce inflammation and promote immune balance
- Probiotics: Support gut health and immune function

- Vitamin D: Regulate immune responses and reduce inflammation
- Turmeric/Curcumin: Potent anti-inflammatory and antioxidant effects
- Ginger: Anti-inflammatory and immune-modulating properties

Supplements for Inflammation Reduction

Discover the benefits of:

- Fish oil supplements
- Probiotic supplements
- Vitamin D supplements
- Turmeric/Curcumin supplements
- Ginger supplements

Tips for Supplementing Your Diet

Ensure safe and effective supplementation:

- Consult with a healthcare professional
- Choose high-quality supplements
- Follow recommended dosages

- Monitor your body's response
- Combine supplements with a balanced diet

The Power of Supplements in Action

By incorporating science-backed supplements, you can:

- Reduce chronic inflammation
- Enhance your immune function
- Improve your overall wellbeing
- Increase your energy levels
- Support your body's natural defenses

Embrace the Supplement Secret

By unlocking the sixth secret of supplements, you'll be empowered to harness the power of science-backed solutions to regulate your immune system and tame inflammation. Remember, supplements are not a replacement for a healthy diet and lifestyle.

Additionally, consider the following:

- Always consult with a healthcare professional before adding new supplements
- Be patient and consistent with supplementation
- Monitor your body's response and adjust your supplement regimen as needed
- Combine supplements with a balanced diet and healthy lifestyle habits
- Stay informed about the latest research and developments in supplement science

Chapter 10: Secret 7: Gut-Friendly Habits for a Balanced Immune System

The Gut-Immune Connection

The gut and immune system are intricately linked. A healthy gut microbiome is essential for a balanced immune system. In this chapter, we'll explore the seventh secret to taming inflammation: gut-friendly habits.

Gut-Friendly Habits for a Balanced Immune System

Discover the power of:

- Fiber-rich foods: Feed good bacteria and promote a balanced gut
- Fermented foods: Support gut health and immune function

- Hydration: Adequate water intake for gut health and immune function
- Stress management: Reduce stress's impact on gut health
- Sleep: Prioritize sleep for gut health and immune function
- Exercise: Regular physical activity for gut health and immune function
- Avoiding antibiotics and antimicrobials: Preserve gut health

The Science Behind Gut-Friendly Habits

Understand the mechanisms:

- Gut barrier function and immune system regulation
- Short-chain fatty acids and immune system modulation
- Gut-brain axis and immune system regulation

Tips for Implementing Gut-Friendly Habits

Start your journey:

- Gradually increase fiber intake
- Incorporate fermented foods into your diet
- Drink plenty of water
- Practice stress-reducing techniques
- Prioritize sleep and aim for 7-9 hours
- Engage in regular physical activity
- Limit antibiotic and antimicrobial use

The Power of Gut-Friendly Habits in Action

By embracing gut-friendly habits, you can:

- Reduce chronic inflammation
- Enhance your immune function
- Improve your overall wellbeing
- Increase your energy levels
- Support your body's natural defenses

Embrace the Gut-Friendly Secret

By unlocking the seventh secret of gut-friendly habits, you'll be empowered to create a balanced immune system and tame inflammation.

Remember, a healthy gut is the foundation of overall well-being.

Additionally, consider the following:

- Be patient and consistent with gut-friendly habits
- Monitor your body's response and adjust your habits as needed
- Combine gut-friendly habits with a balanced diet and healthy lifestyle
- Stay informed about the latest research and developments in gut health and immune function.

PART 3:

PUTTING IT ALL TOGETHER

Chapter 11: Creating Your Personalized Inflammation-Reducing Plan

Tailoring a Plan to Your Needs

Congratulations on completing the 7 secrets to taming inflammation! Now, it's time to create a personalized plan that suits your unique needs and lifestyle.

Assessing Your Inflammation Profile

Reflect on your:

- Diet and nutrition habits
- Stress levels and management techniques
- Sleep quality and duration
- Exercise habits and physical activity

- Gut health and digestive function
- Supplement routine
- Overall health and wellbeing

Setting Realistic Goals and Objectives

Establish achievable goals, such as:

- Reducing body fat percentage
- Improving sleep quality
- Increasing energy levels
- Enhancing mental clarity
- Supporting immune function

Crafting Your Personalized Plan

Combine the 7 secrets to create a tailored plan:

- Nutrition: Incorporate anti-inflammatory foods and supplements
- Stress management: Practice mindfulness, meditation, or yoga
- Sleep: Prioritize 7-9 hours of sleep and establish a relaxing bedtime routine

- Exercise: Engage in regular physical activity, such as walking or swimming
- Gut health: Focus on fiber-rich foods, fermented foods, and probiotics
- Supplements: Consider adding omega-3s, vitamin D, or probiotics
- Mind-body connection: Practice gratitude, journaling, or deep breathing

Monitoring Progress and Adjusting Your Plan

Regularly track your:

- Food intake and nutrition habits
- Stress levels and management techniques
- Sleep quality and duration
- Exercise habits and physical activity
- Gut health and digestive function
- Supplement routine
- Overall health and wellbeing

Embracing a Balanced Lifestyle

Remember, reducing inflammation is a journey. Focus on progress, not perfection. By committing to your personalized plan, you'll be empowered to:

- Reduce chronic inflammation
- Enhance your immune function
- Improve your overall well being
- Increase your energy levels
- Support your body's natural defenses

Celebrate Your Success

Acknowledge and celebrate your achievements along the way. You've taken the first step towards a healthier, happier you!

Chapter 12: Overcoming Common Obstacles and Staying on Track

Embracing the Journey, Not Perfection

Congratulations on creating your personalized inflammation-reducing plan! Now, let's tackle common obstacles that may arise and strategies to stay on track.

Common Obstacles:

1. Lack of motivation: Identify your why and celebrate small victories.

2. Time constraints: Start small, prioritize, and schedule self-care.

3. Social pressures: Communicate your goals, find support, and lead by example.

4. Setbacks: Forgive yourself, learn from mistakes, and move forward.

5. Plateaus: Reassess goals, seek new challenges, and stay patient.

Strategies for Success:

1. Accountability partner: Share goals and progress with a friend or mentor.

2. Tracking progress: Use journals, apps, or spreadsheets to monitor advancements.

3. Reward system: Celebrate milestones with non-food rewards.

4. Mindset shifts: Focus on addition, not subtraction (add healthy habits, don't just remove unhealthy ones).

5. Self-care: Prioritize rest, relaxation, and activities bringing joy.

***Maintaining Momentum*:**

1. Stay informed: Continuously learn about inflammation reduction and overall well-being.

2. Seek support: Join communities, forums, or consult professionals.

3. Be patient: Recognize progress, not perfection.

4. Celebrate milestones: Acknowledge achievements along the way.

5. Stay flexible: Adapt to changes, and adjust your plan as needed.

Overcoming Emotional Eating:

1. Identify triggers: Recognize emotional states leading to unhealthy choices.

2. Find alternative coping mechanisms: Engage in activities bringing comfort and relaxation.

3. Practice mindful eating: Savor food, pay attention to hunger cues, and eat slowly.

Sustaining Long-Term Success:

1. Make it a lifestyle: Incorporate healthy habits into daily routines.

2. Continuously challenge yourself: Set new goals, try new activities, and explore new interests.

3. Stay positive and patient: Focus on progress, not perfection.

By embracing these strategies, you'll be empowered to overcome common obstacles and stay on track with your inflammation-reducing plan, leading to a healthier, happier you!

Chapter 13: Maintaining Momentum and Embracing a Life of Optimal Wellness

Sustaining Progress and Embracing a Wellness Lifestyle

Congratulations on completing your personalized inflammation-reducing plan! Now, let's focus on maintaining momentum and embracing a life of optimal wellness.

Maintaining Momentum:

1. Set new goals: Continuously challenge yourself and set new objectives.

2. Stay accountable: Share progress with a friend or mentor and track advancements.

3.   Celebrate   milestones: Acknowledge achievements along the way.

4. Stay informed: Continuously learn about inflammation reduction and overall well-being.

5. Seek support: Join communities, forums, or consult professionals.

Embracing a Wellness Lifestyle:

1. Make it a habit: Incorporate healthy habits into daily routines.

2. Find activities you enjoy: Engage in physical activities and hobbies that bring joy.

3. Prioritize self-care: Focus on rest, relaxation, and stress management.

4. Nurture relationships: Surround yourself with supportive people.

5. Stay positive and patient: Focus on progress, not perfection.

The Power of Mindset:

1. Growth mindset: Embrace challenges and view failures as opportunities.

2. Positive self-talk: Encourage yourself with positive affirmations.

3. Self-compassion: Treat yourself with kindness and understanding.

4. Resilience: Develop coping strategies and bounce back from setbacks.

5. Gratitude: Focus on the present and express gratitude for life's blessings.

Embracing a Life of Optimal Wellness:

1. Integrate healthy habits: Make wellness a part of your daily life.

2. Find purpose and meaning: Engage in activities bringing fulfillment.

3. Nurture your spirit: Prioritize self-care, mindfulness, and connection.

4. Stay curious and open-minded: Continuously learn and explore new experiences.

5. Radiate positivity and kindness: Share your energy with others.

By maintaining momentum and embracing a life of optimal wellness, you'll unlock a journey of continuous growth, self-discovery, and vibrant health. Remember, wellness is a journey, not a destination.

CONCLUSION

Empowered and in Control: Your Journey to a Life Beyond Inflammation

Congratulations on Your Journey!

You've completed the 7 secrets to taming inflammation and created a personalized plan to reduce inflammation and improve your overall well-being. This journey has empowered you with knowledge, strategies, and tools to take control of your health.

Reflection and Celebration

Reflect on your journey:

- Celebrate your successes and progress

- Acknowledge challenges and lessons learned
- Recognize your growth and newfound empowerment

Embracing Your New Lifestyle

Remember, this journey is not a destination, but a continuous path to wellness:

- Stay committed to your plan and habits
- Continuously learn and adapt to new information
- Share your knowledge and inspire others

The Power of Empowerment

You now possess the power to:

- Reduce inflammation and improve overall health
- Make informed decisions about your wellbeing
- Take control of your life and choices
- Inspire others to embark on their journey

A Life Beyond Inflammation

Envision your life beyond inflammation:

- Vibrant health and energy
- Clarity of mind and purpose
- Resilience and adaptability
- Meaningful relationships and connections
- A life of purpose and fulfillment

Stay Empowered, Stay in Control

Remember, your journey is unique, and your path to wellness is yours alone. Stay empowered, stay in control, and continue to thrive on your journey to a life beyond inflammation.

Final Thoughts

- You've taken the first step towards a life of optimal wellness
- Continue to nurture your body, mind, and spirit
- Share your journey and inspire others to take control of their health

- Stay curious, stay open-minded, and stay empowered

Congratulations on completing your journey to a life beyond inflammation!

APPENDIX

Additional Resources for Further Learning

Books:

1. "The Anti-Inflammatory Diet" by Dr. Andrew Weil
2. "The Inflammation Solution" by Dr. William Davis
3. "The Gut-Brain Axis" by Dr. David Perlmutter

Online Courses:

1. "Inflammation and Chronic Disease" on Coursera

2. "Nutrition and Wellness" on edX
3. "Mindfulness and Stress Reduction" on Udemy

Websites:

1. The National Institutes of Health (NIH) - (link unavailable)
2. The Academy of Nutrition and Dietetics - (link unavailable)
3. The Mindfulness Project - (link unavailable)

Podcasts:

1. "The Model Health Show" with Shawn Stevenson
2. "The Mindful Kind" with Rachael Kable
3. "The Nutrition Diva" with Monica Reinagel

Videos:

1. "The Inflammation Documentary" on YouTube
2. "The Gut-Brain Connection" on TED Talks

3. "Mindfulness and Meditation" on Vimeo

Communities:

1. The Inflammation Support Group on Facebook
2. The Mindfulness Community on Reddit
3. The Nutrition and Wellness Forum on Quora

Apps:

1. Headspace for meditation and mindfulness
2. MyFitnessPal for nutrition tracking
3. Fitbit Coach for personalized workouts

Healthcare Professionals:

1. Find a registered dietitian (RD) or registered dietitian nutritionist (RDN) in your area
2. Consult with a healthcare provider or functional medicine doctor
3. Seek guidance from a licensed therapist or counselor

Remember, knowledge is power. Continuously educate yourself and stay updated on the latest research and findings to optimize your journey to a life beyond inflammation.

Glossary of Key Terms

Anti-Inflammatory: Refers to substances or processes that reduce or counteract inflammation.

Chronic Inflammation: Ongoing, low-grade inflammation that persists over time, contributing to various diseases.

Cytokines: Signaling molecules that facilitate communication between immune cells, influencing inflammation.

Gut-Brain Axis: The bidirectional relationship between the gut microbiome and the central nervous system.

Inflammation: The body's natural response to injury or infection, characterized by increased blood flow, swelling, and immune cell activation.

Mind-Body Connection: The intricate relationship between mental and emotional states and physical wellbeing.

Omega-3 Fatty Acids: Essential fatty acids, particularly EPA and DHA, that reduce inflammation and promote heart health.

Oxidative Stress: Imbalance between free radicals and antioxidants, leading to cellular damage and inflammation.

Probiotics: Live microorganisms that confer health benefits, particularly in the gut microbiome.

Stress Response: The body's reaction to stress, involving the hypothalamic-pituitary-adrenal (HPA) axis and cortisol release.

Turmeric/Curcumin: A spice and its active compound, respectively, with potent anti-inflammatory and antioxidant properties.

Vitamin D: A fat-soluble vitamin essential for immune regulation, bone health, and inflammation reduction.

Wellness: A state of optimal physical, mental, and emotional health, encompassing lifestyle choices and self-care practices.

By familiarizing yourself with these key terms, you'll deepen your understanding of the complex relationships between inflammation, lifestyle, and overall well-being.